W9-BMY-012

THE DAY I MET
THE NUTS

Spencer, Riley, and Kaylin ~
With warm wishes,
Mary Rand Hess

OK,
NO
NUTS

by Mary Rand Hess
Illustrated by Candice Hartsough McDonald

Earth Day Publishing
Virginia

Publisher's Cataloging-in-Publication
(Provided by Quality Books, Inc.)

Hess, Mary Rand.
  The day I met the nuts / by Mary Rand Hess ;
illustrated by Candice Hartsough McDonald.
    p. cm.
    SUMMARY: A young boy attends a birthday party and has
an allergic reaction to the nut-filled birthday cake. A
doctor treats him with a shot and tells him he must stay
away from all nuts. The child is upset since many of his
favorite foods contain traces of nuts. However, he and
his mother discover plenty of other good foods at the
grocery store and, the next day at school, he starts the
"no nuts allowed" club at the nut-free cafeteria table.
    Audience: Grades Pre-K through 3.
    ISBN-13: 978-0-9842178-0-9 (hardcover)
    ISBN-10: 0-9842178-0-0 (hardcover)
    ISBN-13: 978-0-9842178-1-6 (paperback)
    ISBN-10: 0-9842178-1-9 (paperback.)

    1. Food allergy--Juvenile fiction. 2. Nut--Juvenile
fiction. 3. Nut products--Juvenile fiction. 4. Food
allergy--Diet therapy--Juvenile fiction. [1. Food
allergy--Fiction. 2. Nut--Fiction. 3. Food allergy--
Diet therapy--Fiction.]   I. McDonald, Candice
Hartsough, 1982- ill. II. Title.

PZ7.H4356Day 2009   [E]
            QBI09-600148

Published by EARTH DAY PUBLISHING
Copyright © 2009 by Earth Day Publishing, LLC
All rights reserved. For information about permission to reproduce
selections from this book, address: Book Editor,
Earth Day Publishing, P.O. Box 650543,
Potomac Falls, VA 20165-0543

www.earthdaypublishing.com

Book design by Amber Leberman

The text of this book is set in Adobe Garamond Pro.
The illustrations are done in watercolor, colored pencil, and graphite.

Printed in the United States of America

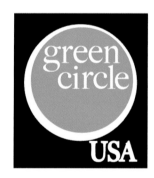

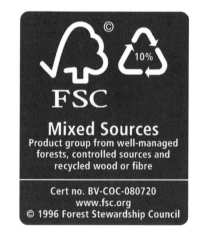

ECO-FRIENDLY BOOKS
Made in the USA

To Roman and Trenton, my allergy champions—
I love you.
~M.R.H

For all the teachers who believed in me.
~C.H.M

I was at my best friend's
birthday party when it happened.

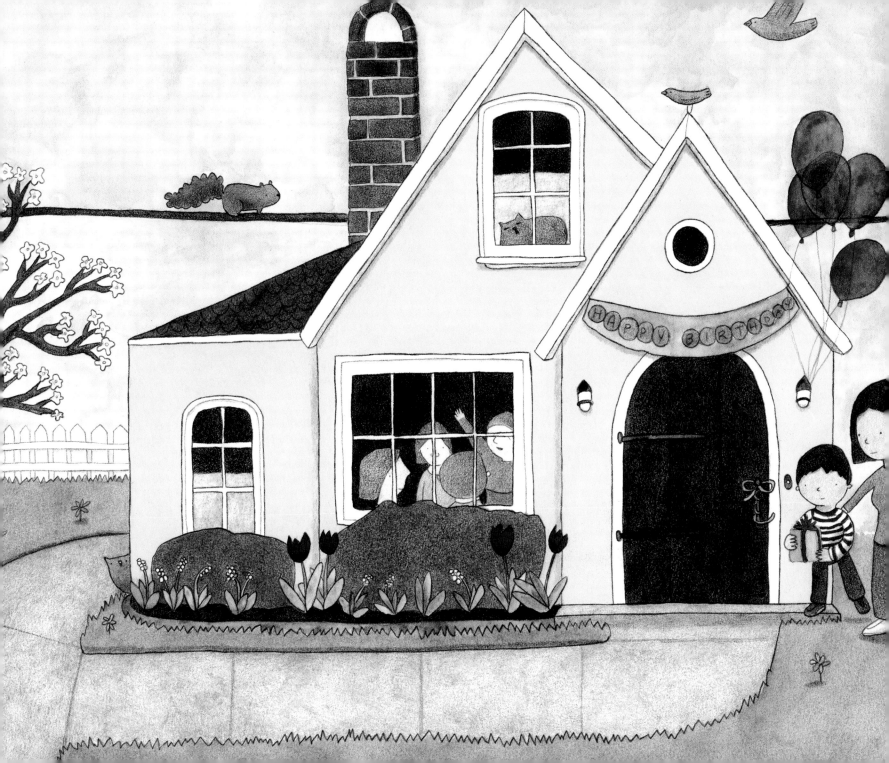

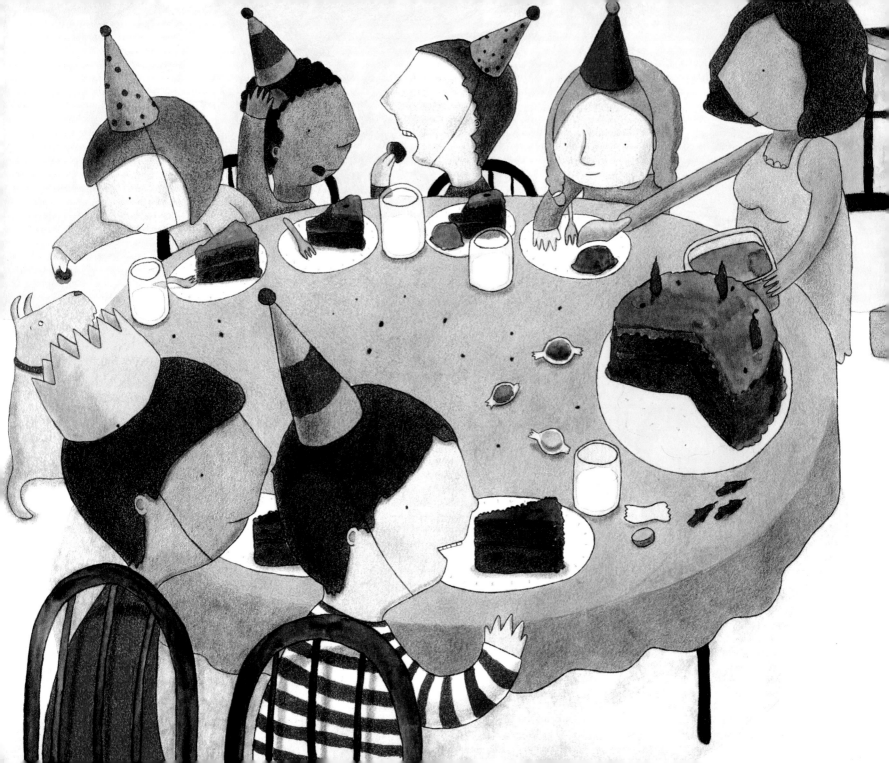

The birthday song was sung in high gear. Secret wishes were made. Candles were blown out.

Then the birthday cake was served.

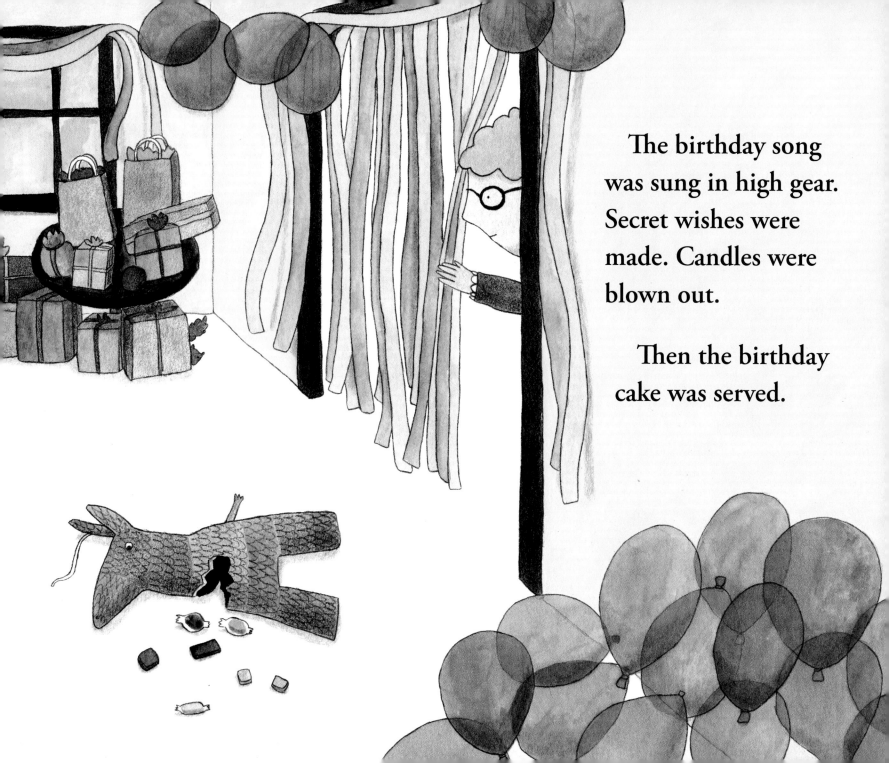

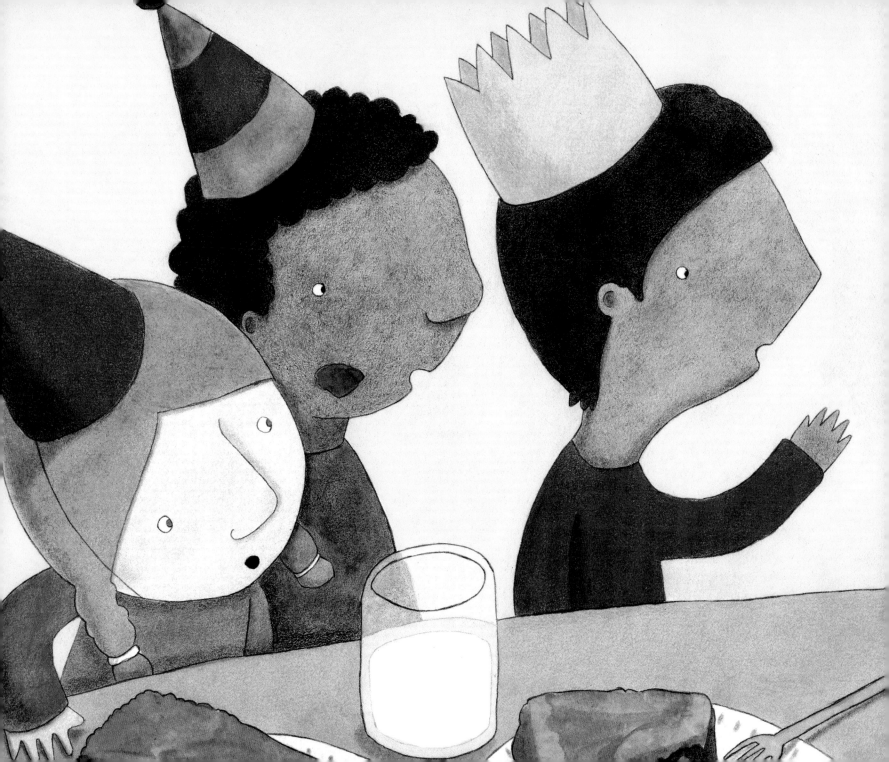

We dug into our *double chocolate muddy-nutty cake*. I took two bites and The Nuts attacked me like wild fire ants. I itched and I scratched, and the madness made me quite mad. That's when Mom rushed me over for a visit with Doctor McFever.

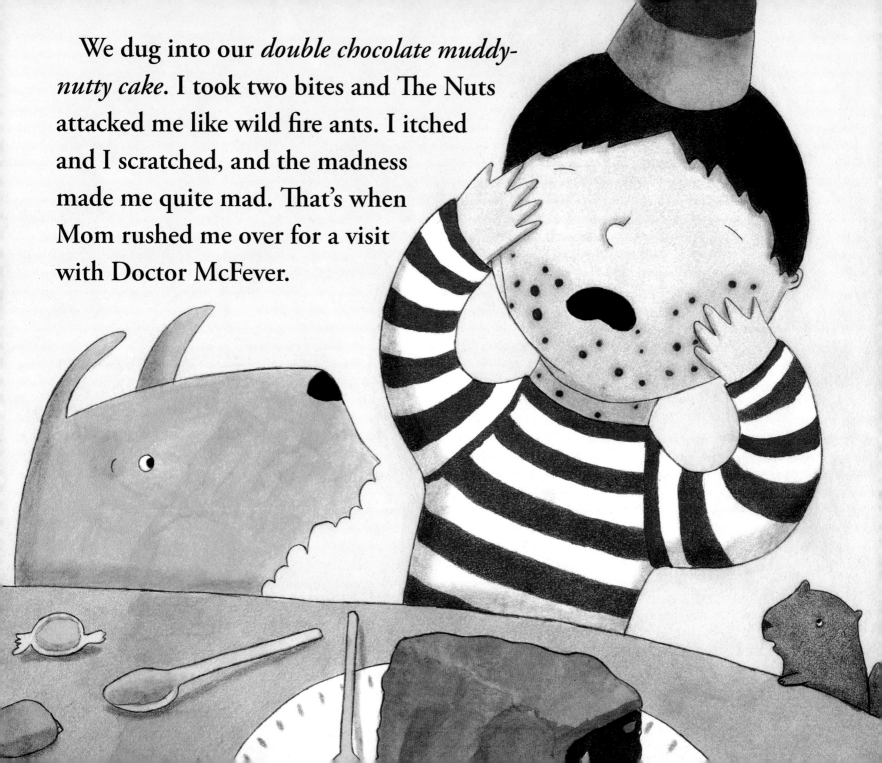

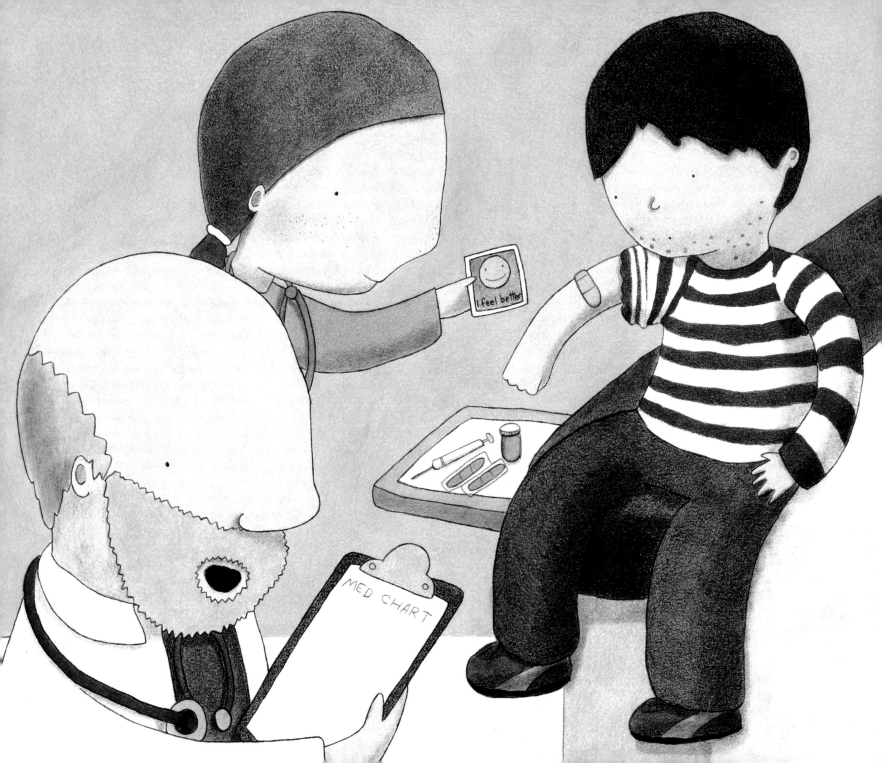

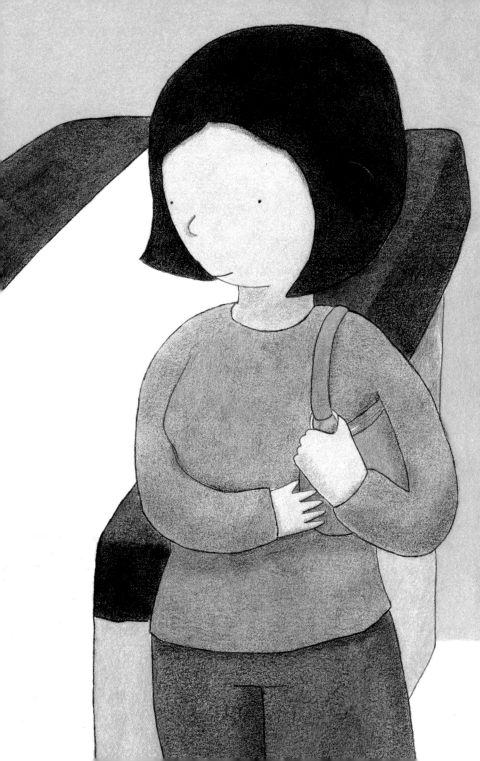

The nurse and doctor greeted me right away. They gave me a shot in my arm. The shot stung a little, but it made the mad itching stop.

"Stay away from NUTS!" Dr. McFever said.

"You + nuts = disaster."

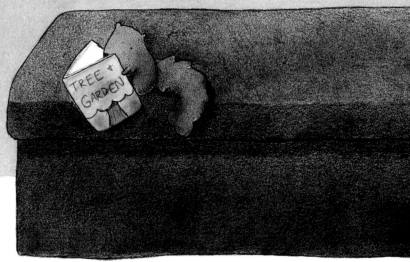

"Why don't nuts like me?" I asked.

"It's really YOUR body that doesn't like nuts. You're better off without them. Each time you eat something with nuts, your reaction could get worse."

"Will The Nuts and I ever get along?" I asked.

"I don't know for sure. But until we can find away for you and The Nuts to be friends, you will need to keep special medicine nearby just in case. So for now, NO NUTTING AROUND!" Dr. McFever said.

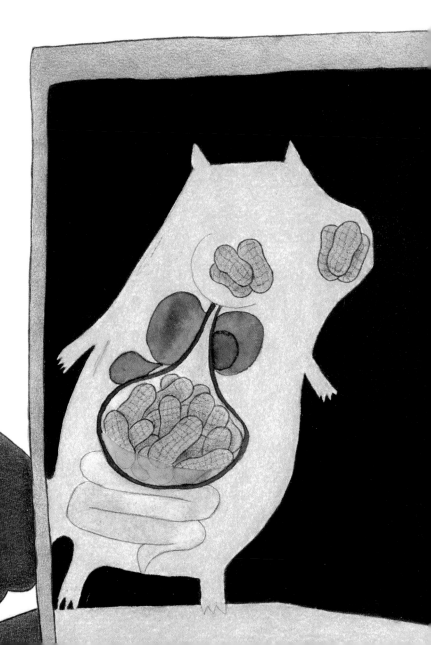

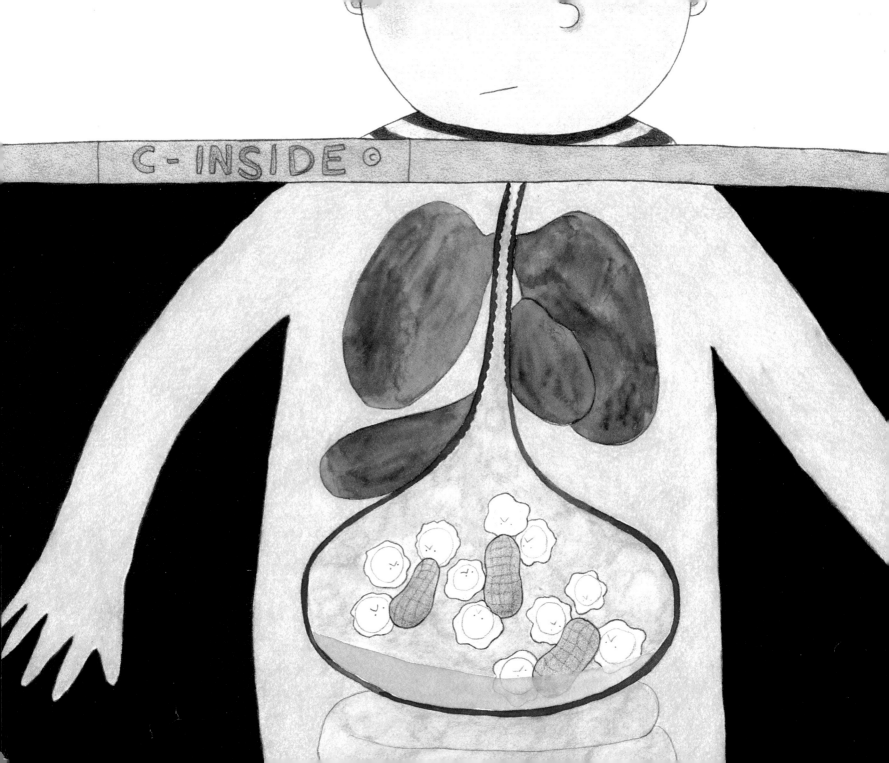

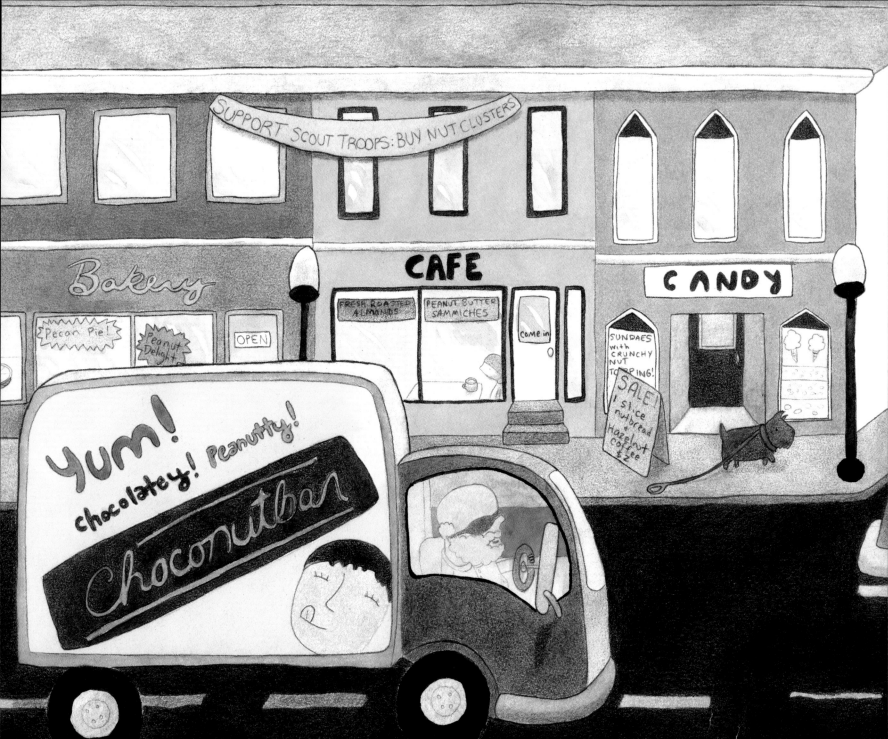

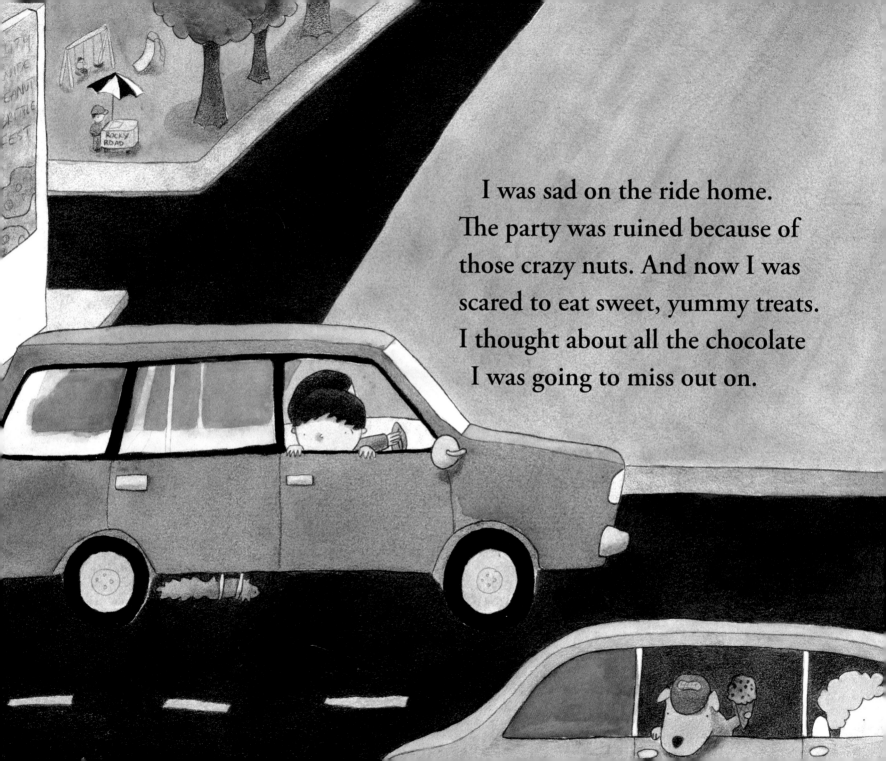

I was sad on the ride home. The party was ruined because of those crazy nuts. And now I was scared to eat sweet, yummy treats. I thought about all the chocolate I was going to miss out on.

I thought of Pecans dancing on top of chocolate pies.
Almonds jumping for joy. Peanuts snickering at me.
Cashews making me ACHOO.
Walnuts driving me up the wall.

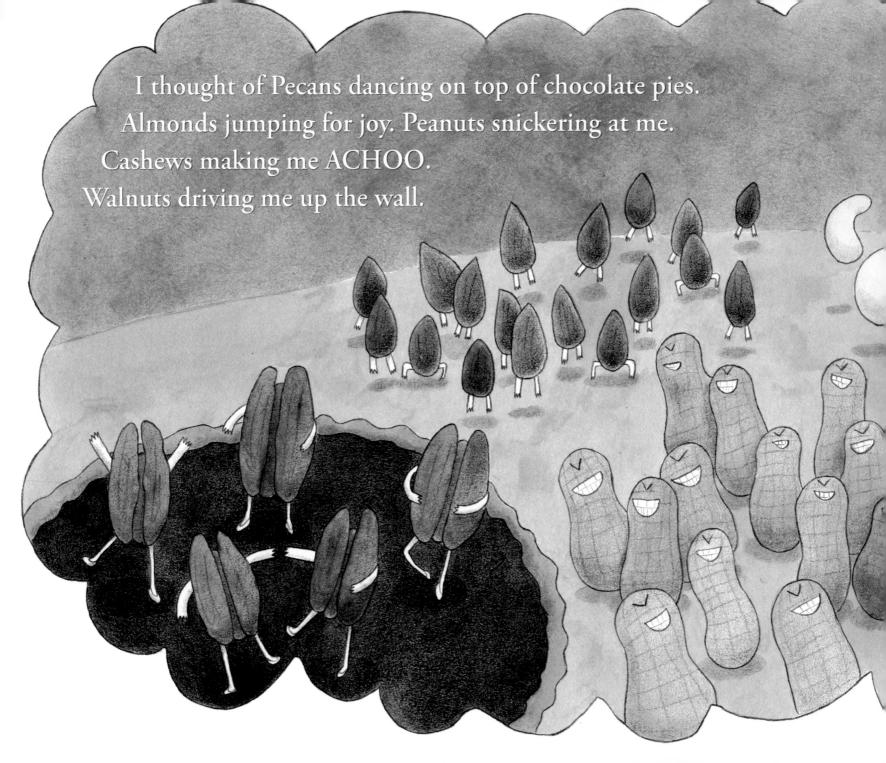

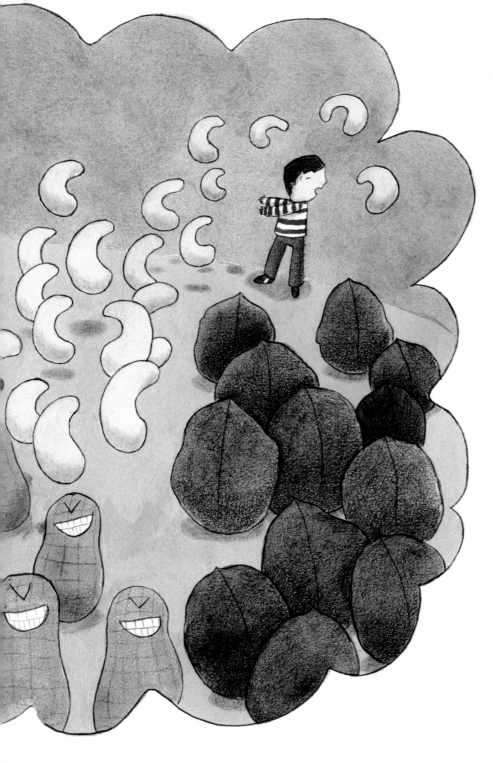

Mom said all would be okay.
"We will adjust," she said.
I'm not sure what adjust means,
but I don't ever want to itch
like that again.

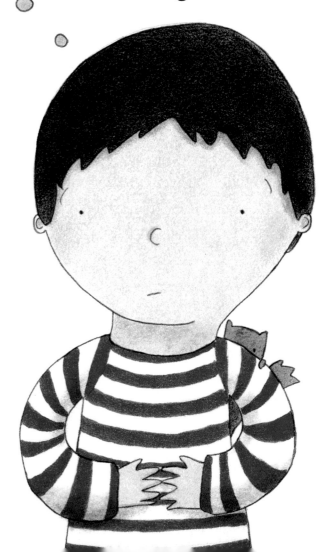

When I got home, I took my hamster, Peanut, out of his cage. Right then and there, we decided to change his name to French Fry. Mom, French Fry, and I went through the pantry. We looked at all the labels on boxes, bags, and cans.

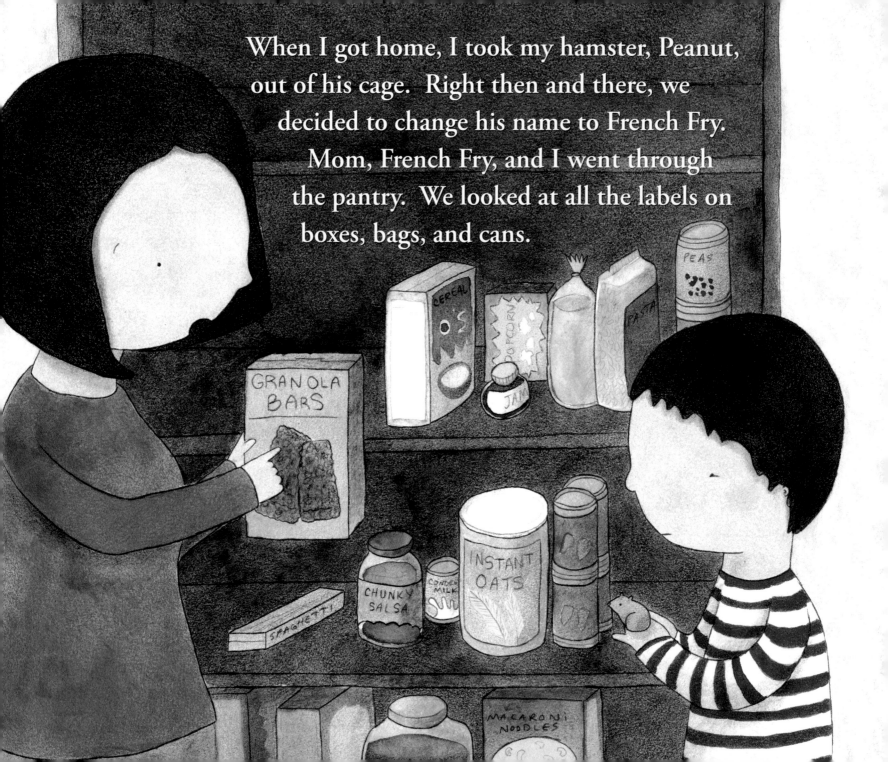

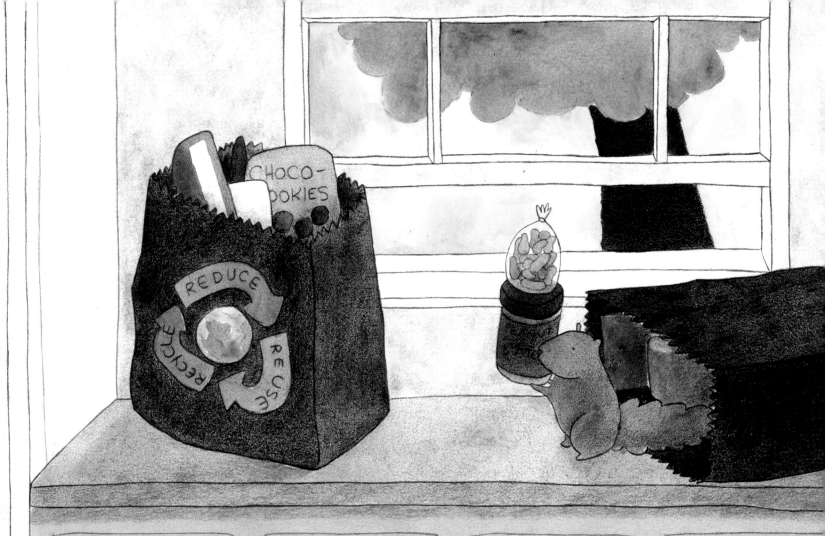

May contain traces of nuts. Manufactured on shared equipment that processes nuts. Contains nuts!

We bagged all the groceries that contained or may contain nuts. We set them aside for the next food drive.

"Good bye, nuts!" I shouted. But it's not that easy I found out.

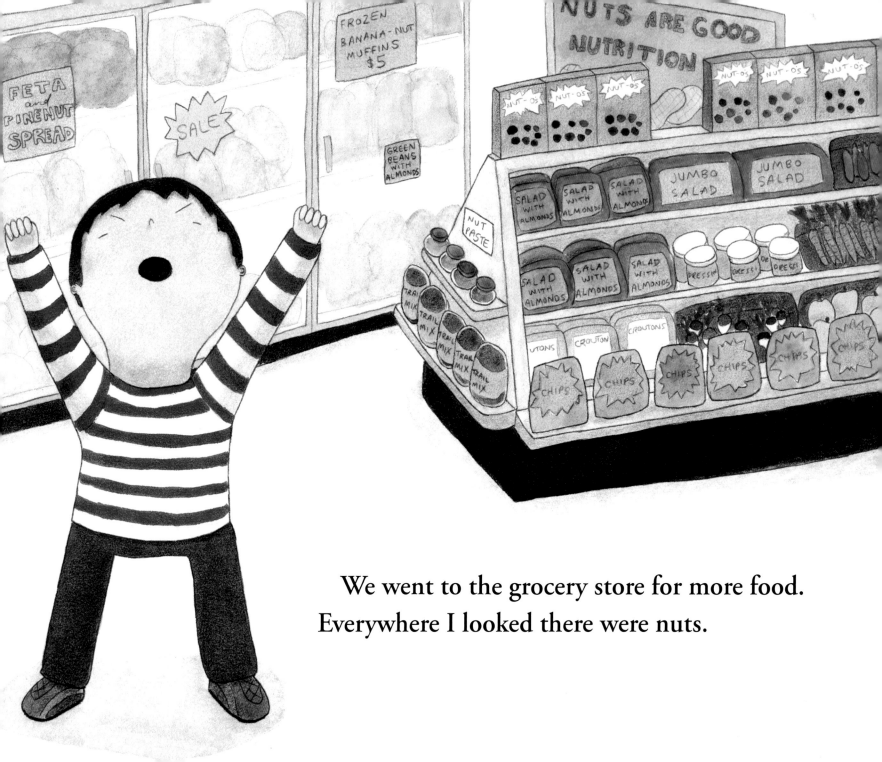

We went to the grocery store for more food.
Everywhere I looked there were nuts.

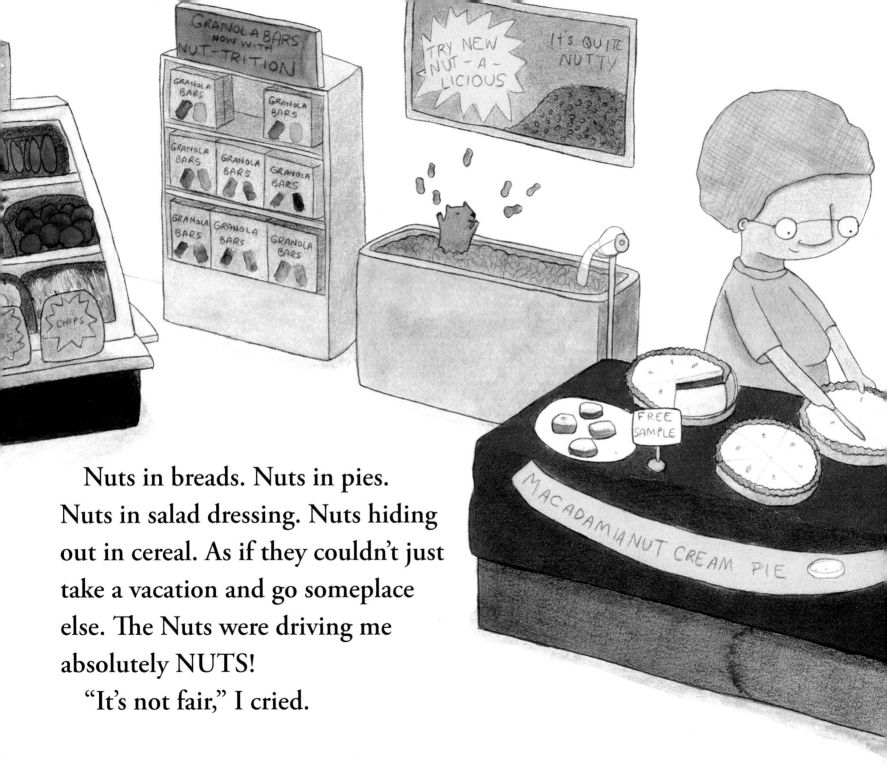

Nuts in breads. Nuts in pies. Nuts in salad dressing. Nuts hiding out in cereal. As if they couldn't just take a vacation and go someplace else. The Nuts were driving me absolutely NUTS!

"It's not fair," I cried.

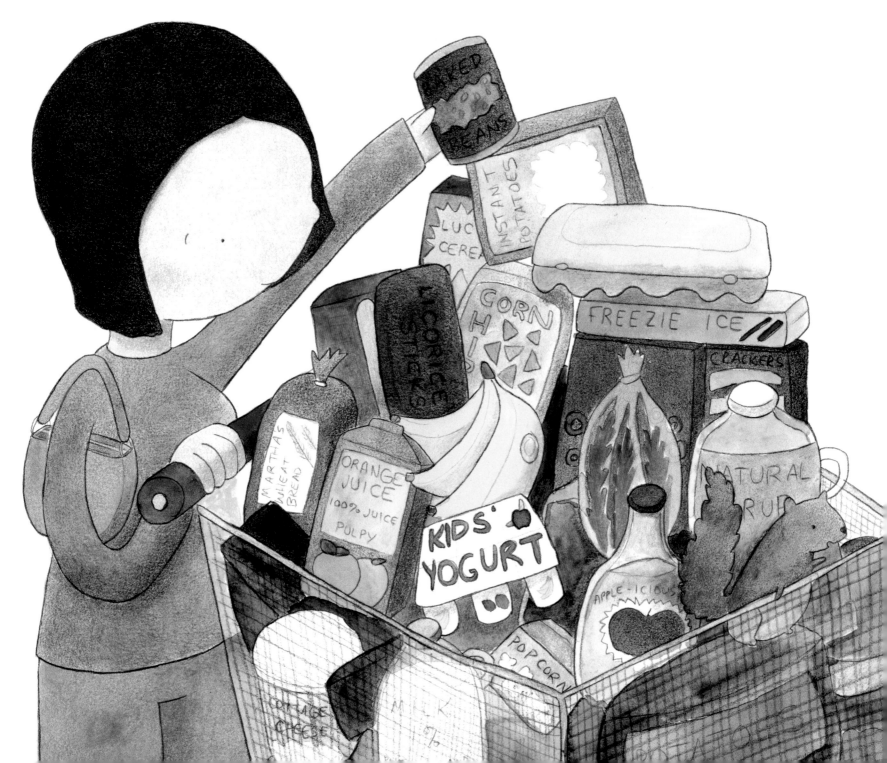

But Mom showed me there's enough good food in the world for us all. And to prove it, our cart was soon piled high, even with a little chocolate that was safe to eat.

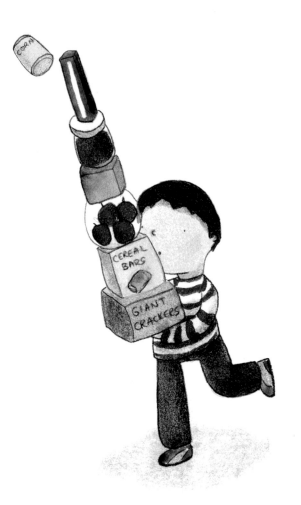

We put our groceries on the belt. I loaded on the bananas.
"I can't believe I'm allergic to nuts," I said to the cashier.
"Nuts are nutty sometimes," he said.
That's when the kid behind me announced, "Well, I'm allergic to bananas. They drive me absolutely bananas!"

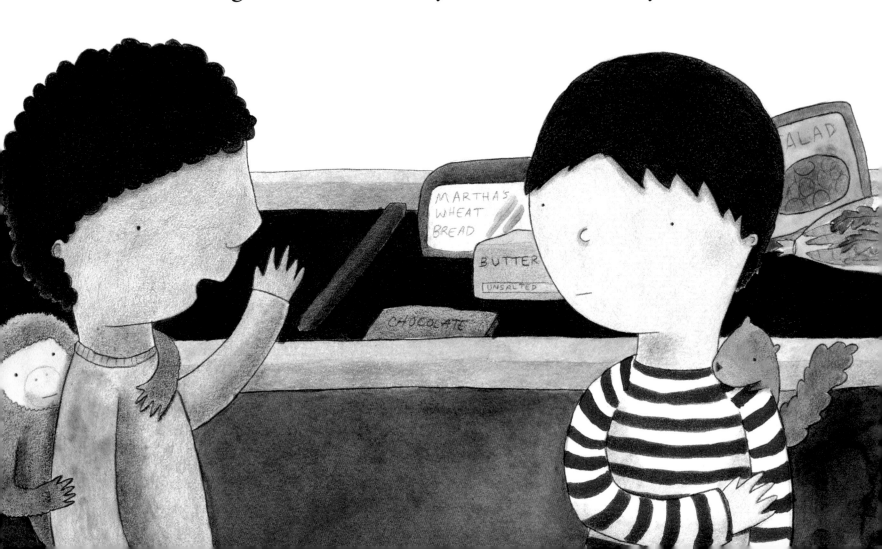

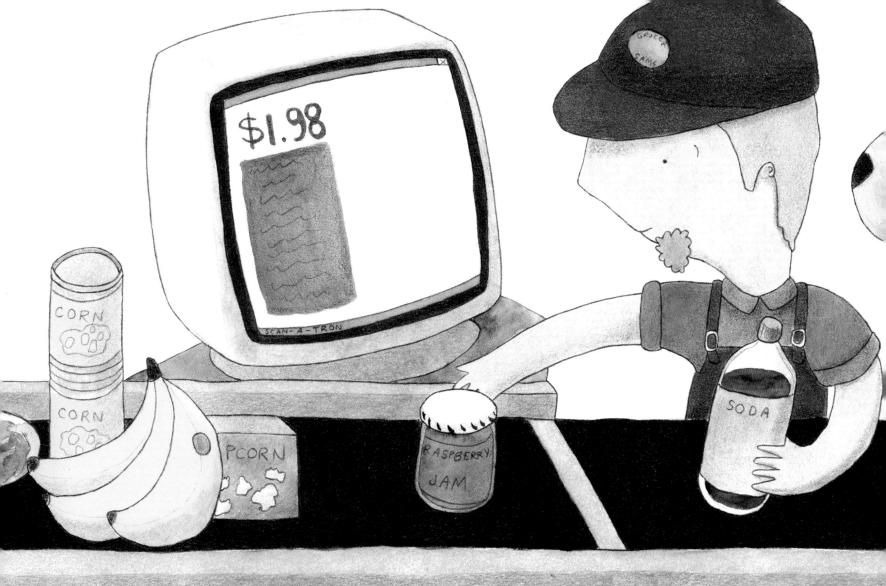

"Wow! I'm not alone," I said. "I thought I was the only one allergic to something as nutty as nuts or as crazy as bananas."
The kid and I exchanged high-fives.

The cashier chimed in...
"And I'm allergic to blackberries.
Berries make me berry mad."

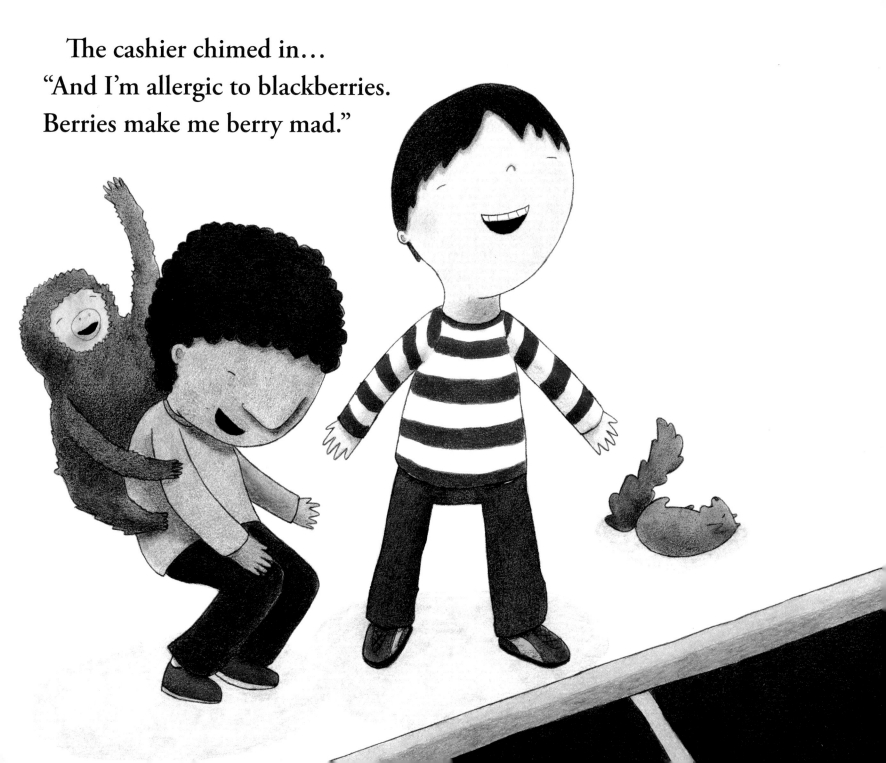

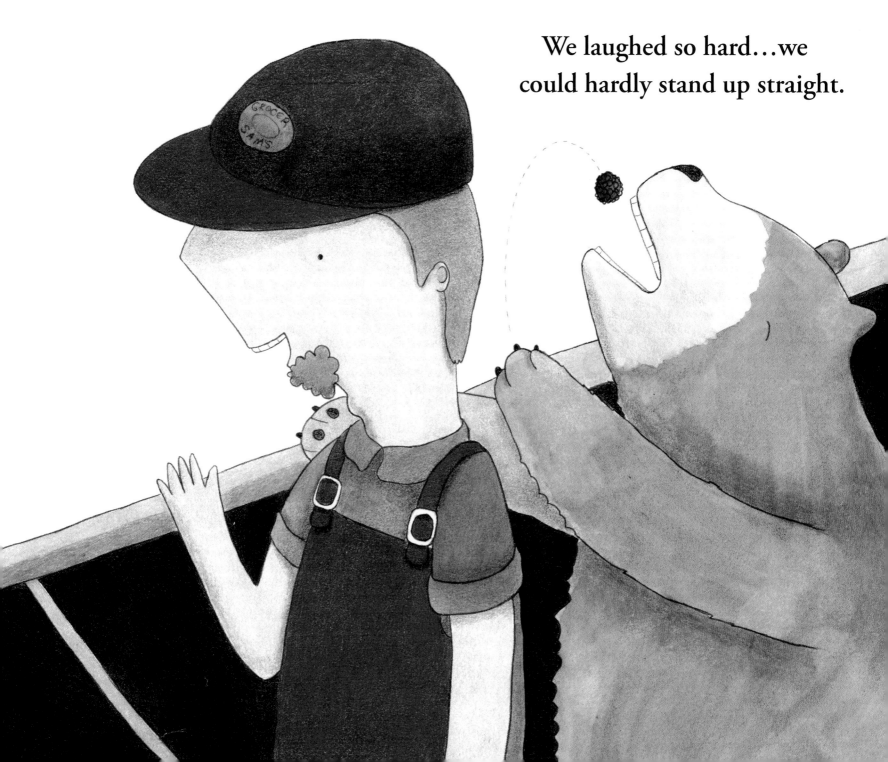

We laughed so hard…we could hardly stand up straight.

During dinner that night, Mom and
I told the family our pre-dic-a-ment.
Another big word I learned.

"No nuts are allowed in this house,"
I announced to Dad, my brother, and
my sister.

They all got up from their chairs to
give me big bear hugs, because they
knew it had been a rough day.

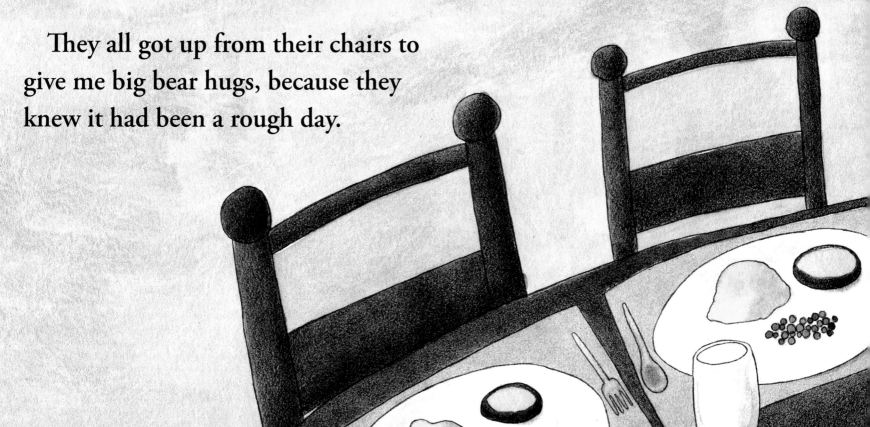

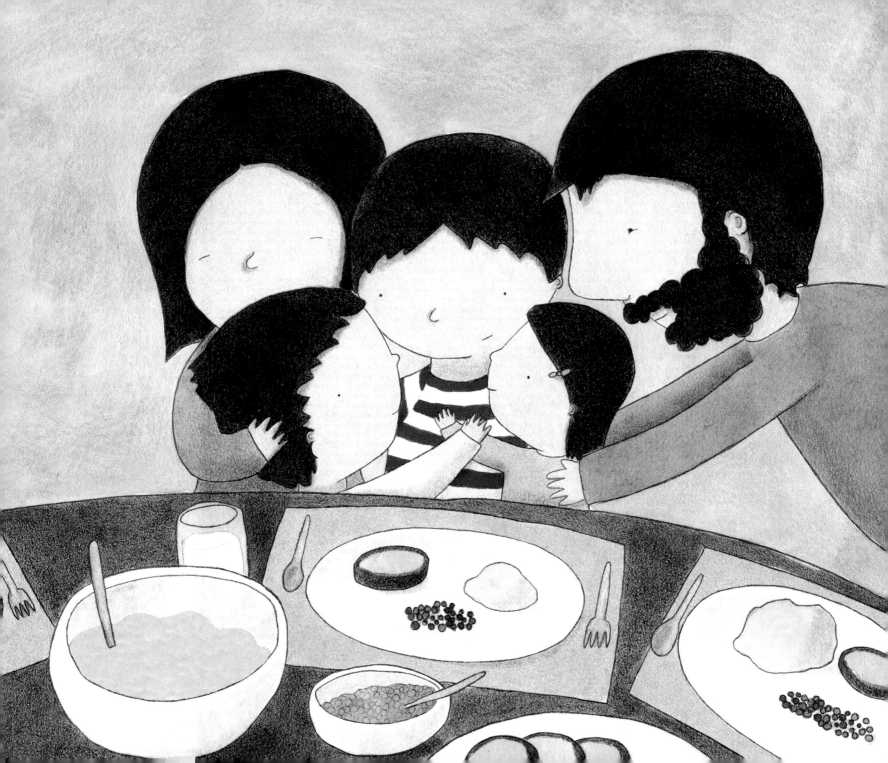

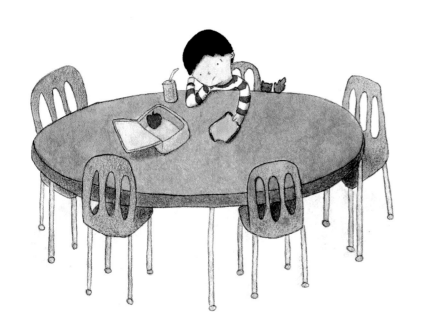

The next afternoon at lunch, my teacher pointed to a table at the back of the cafeteria.

"It's a NUT FREE table for you and any others who are allergic to nuts," she said.

I walked over to the table. No one was there. I sat down…all alone. I was sad thinking that I might be eating lunch by myself for the rest of my life, and all because I met The Nuts.

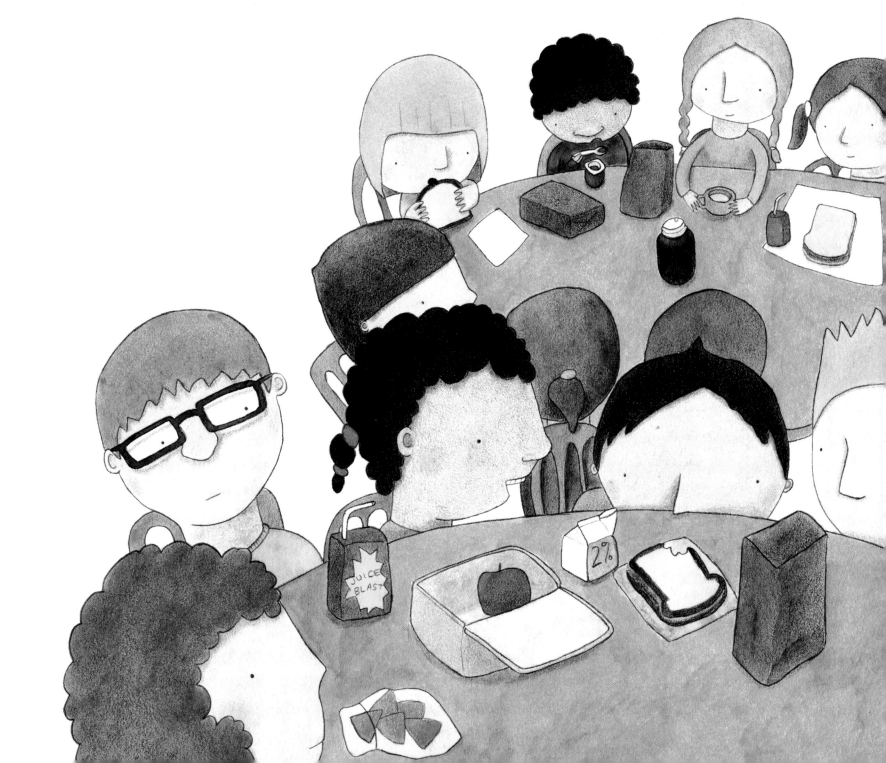

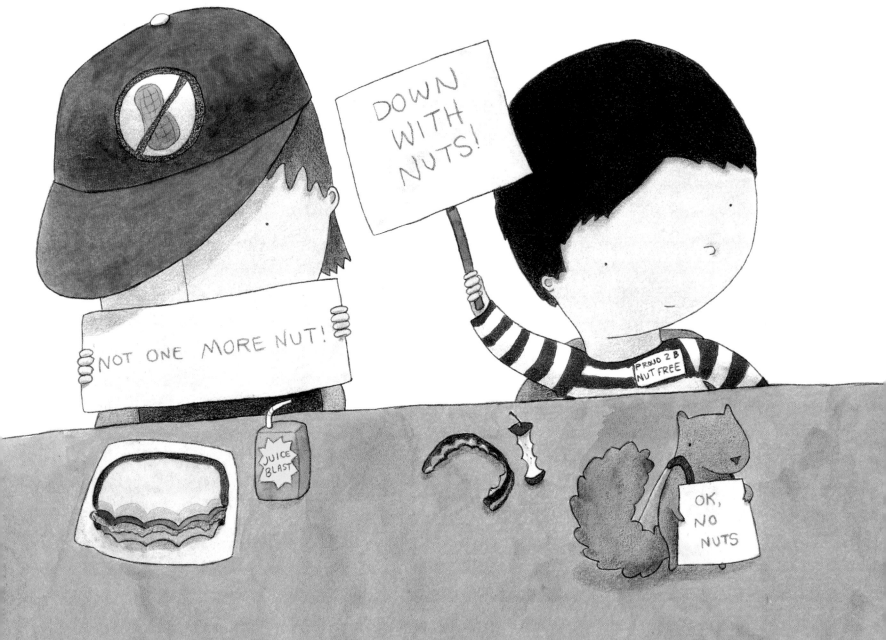

But before I knew it, some of my friends, and other kids I didn't even know, came to sit with me. We formed a NO NUTS ALLOWED club.

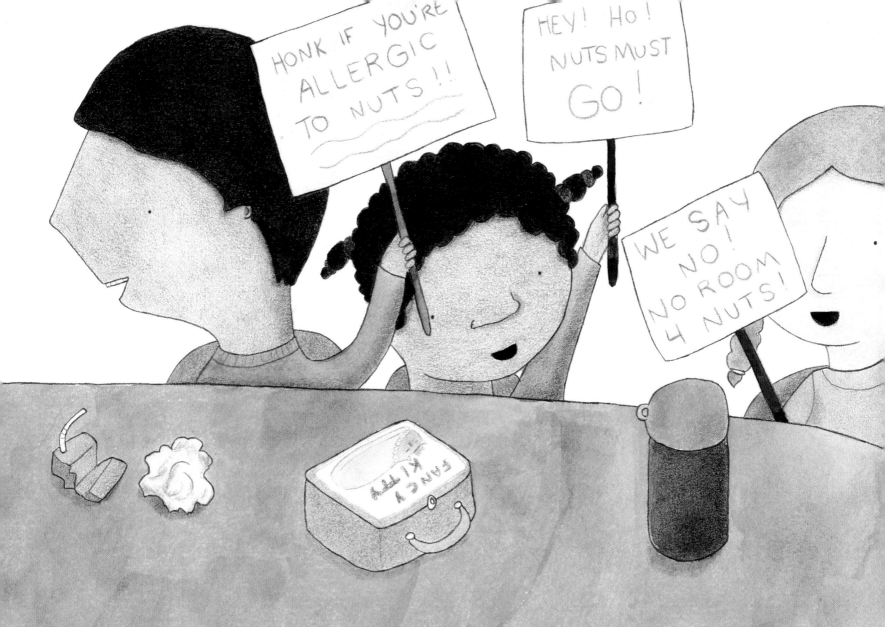

You don't have to be allergic to nuts to join, but you CANNOT bring nuts with you. Nuts are outlawed here!

The day I met The Nuts changed everything. I made new friends, have a cool club, and I can even read some big words now.

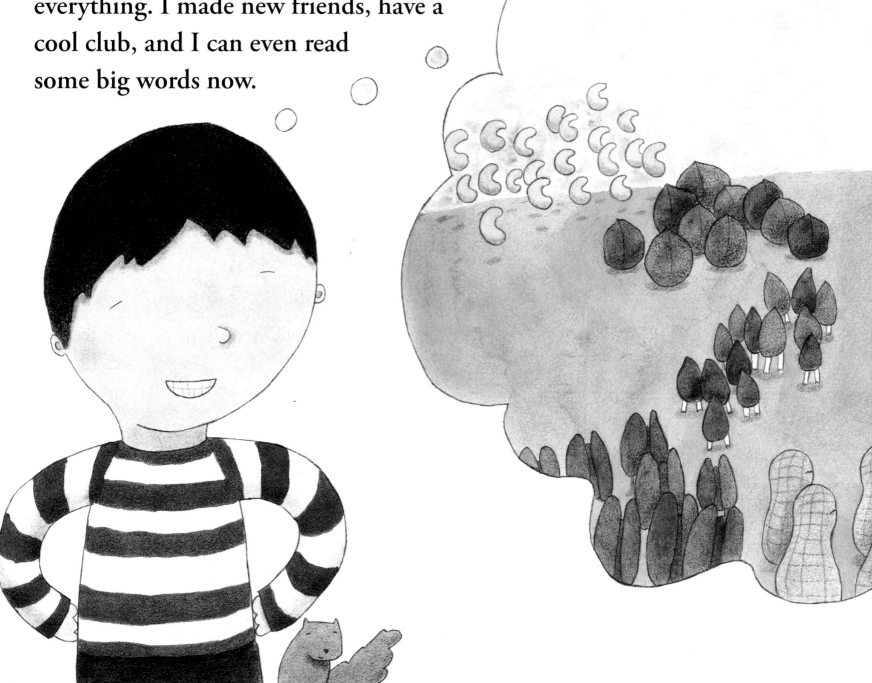

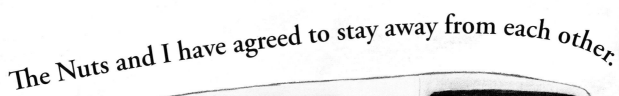

The Nuts and I have agreed to stay away from each other.

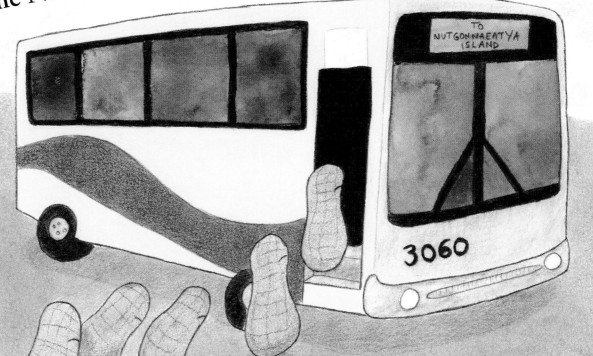

No pecans dancing on top of chocolate pies. No peanuts snickering at me. No cashews making me ACHOO. No walnuts driving me up the wall. Just me going NUT FREE! And I feel good.

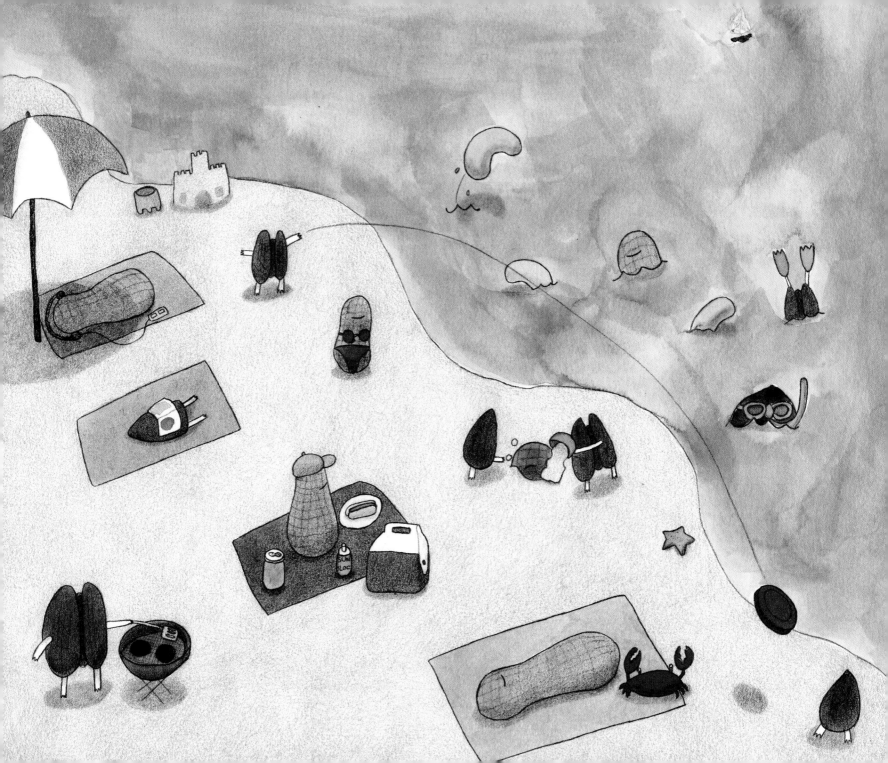

Mary Rand Hess

Mary Rand Hess writes for children and young adults. She gets much of her inspiration from her two sons and the students she meets while teaching creative writing. When she's not busy dreaming up stories, she loves to compose music on the piano, dance, bake, and travel with her family. Oh and by the way, she is also allergic to The Nuts.

www.maryrandhess.com

Candice Hartsough McDonald

Candice Hartsough McDonald was born in a midsized Midwestern city. One day she was given some crayons to color with, and she has never stopped. Her adventures include graduating from the Herron School of Art and Design in Indianapolis, Indiana, taking part in art exhibitions across the city and beyond, raising a fine young kitty named Mona, and marrying her best friend, Brandon. She lives in Indianapolis.

www.cordialkitten.com

Did you know?

Approximately 12 million Americans have food allergies. More than three million of those people are allergic to nuts and many of them are children. Those who are allergic to foods must often carry around special medicine like epinephrine just in case of a severe reaction.

Much research is being done to help find a cure for food allergies. With the support of parents, schools, doctors, pharmacists, and charitable organizations, we can find a way.

Earth Day Publishing

Earth Day Publishing supports organizations that increase awareness and improve our health, the environment, and education.

To find out more about the organizations we support and to be a part of our mission, visit us at **www.earthdaypublishing.com**.